DIABETES

HOW TO HELP

EVERYTHING YOU NEED TO KNOW ABOUT DIABETES TYPE 1 AND TYPE 2

Dr. Robertino Bedenian

Diabetes How to Help: Everything You Need to Know About Diabetes Type 1 and Type 2

Dr. Robertino Bedenian

Published by Dr. Robertino Bedenian, 2024.

DIABETES HOW TO HELP: EVERYTHING YOU NEED TO KNOW ABOUT DIABETES TYPE 1 AND TYPE 2

First edition. February 3, 2024.

Copyright © 2024 Dr. Robertino Bedenian.

ISBN: 979-8223697732

Written by Dr. Robertino Bedenian.

Also by Dr. Robertino Bedenian

Fitness Over 60 For Women – How to Stay Fit And Healthy As You Age

Does Back Pain Go Away? 10 Answers To The Most Acute Back Pain Issues

Massage Bible - A Beginners Guide To Western And Eastern Massage Therapy

Going Vegan - How To Vegan Without Going Crazy

Chiropraktik - Was Steckt Eigentlich Dahinter?

Massagen: Ein Überblick Über Westliche Und Östliche Massagetechniken

Natuerlich Abnehmen, Schlank Und Endlich Fit Sein

P.S. Ich Liebe Dich: Wenn Liebe So Einfach Wäre

Was Tun Bei Rückenschmerzen, Bandscheibenvorfall Und Ischiasschmerzen: 10 Antworten Zu Den Häufigsten Fragen Bei Rückenschmerzen

Was Tun Gegen Schlafapnoe, Schlafstörungen Und Schnarchen

Self-Help Books for Women – How to Overcome Depression, Anxiety, Divorce, Addiction, and Trauma

Diabetes How to Help: Everything You Need to Know About Diabetes Type 1 and Type 2

Diet and Workout Planner: How to Stay Healthy and Get Fit for Life

Everything I Know About Love

The Sleep Easy Solution Book: How to Stop Sleep Apnea, Snoring, and Sleep Disorders

Your Super Gut Feeling Restored – How to Restore Your Life Energy and Overall Health from The Inside Out

Watch for more at https://booksummarypublishing.com.

Table of Contents

Chapter 1: Introduction to Diabetes

Diabetes is a chronic (long-lasting) health condition that affects how your body turns food into energy. Most of the food you eat is broken down into sugar (also called glucose) and released into your bloodstream. When your blood sugar goes up, it signals your pancreas to release insulin.

According to the Center for Disease Control (CDC)

"Diabetes Mellitus (often known as "diabetes") is a dangerous disease in which your body has trouble controlling the quantity of dissolved sugar (glucose) in your bloodstream."

Diabetes is also referred to as "a touch of sugar" or "borderline diabetes." These words imply that someone does not have diabetes or has a milder form of the disease. Diabetes affected 34,2 million persons in the United States in 2020, accounting for almost 10% of the population. More than one-fourth of them were unaware that they suffered from this health issue. One in four people over the age of 65 has diabetes. In adults, Type 2 diabetes accounts for 90-95 percent of occurrences.

Difference between Diabetes Mellitus and Diabetes Insipidus

Diabetes insipidus I is often confused with diabetes mellitus. The two illnesses are unconnected, with diabetes insipidus being an entirely distinct disease. Diabetes mellitus, on the other hand, is significantly more frequent.

Diabetes Mellitus is unrelated to an illness with the same name, "Diabetes Insipidus," which causes fluid retention in the kidneys.

Diabetes insipidus and diabetes mellitus are not the same things. Both illnesses can increase thirst, beverage intake, and urine, but they are unrelated. The level of glucose in your blood, commonly known as blood sugar, is too high in diabetes mellitus. The word 'diabetes' comes from a Greek word that means 'siphon' or 'go 'through.' It means that diabetes mellitus and insipidus are uncontrolled alluding to the production of a large amount of urine.

Insulin resistance or deficiency leads to diabetes mellitus, which is characterized by elevated blood glucose levels.

Diabetes Insipidus, on the other hand, is caused by a halt in the synthesis of a hormone released by the brain to prevent the kidneys from generating too much urine in order to retain water. Water is not retained without this hormone, and the kidneys are always working at maximum capacity.

The term "Mellitus" is a reference to the high levels of sugar in the blood and derives from an old word that roughly translates to "to sweeten with honey." Insipidus, on the other hand, means "unpalatable" and is used to define a type of diabetes that does not cause high blood sugar levels.

Symptoms of Each

Although the symptoms of diabetes mellitus and diabetes insipidus are similar, the causes of these symptoms are different.

Exhaustion

If you have diabetes insipidus, you may have acute exhaustion as a result of dehydration. It could also be due to a deficiency in electrolytes like salt, potassium, or calcium, which are flushed out with all that urine.

When your blood sugar level is either low or too high, you may feel extremely exhausted if you have diabetes.

Thirst

Diabetes insipidus makes you thirsty since your body is losing so much fluid. You become thirsty if you have diabetes mellitus, which is caused by an excess of glucose in your blood. To flush away the sugar, your body needs you to drink more water.

Role of Insulin and Glucose in Diabetes Mellitus

Insulin, a hormone produced by the pancreas, aids glucose absorption into cells for energy use. Sometimes your body doesn't produce enough or any insulin, or it doesn't use it properly. Glucose remains in your circulation and does not reach your cells as a result.

Having too much glucose in your blood might lead to health issues over time. To comprehend diabetes, one must first comprehend the role of glucose in the body, as well as what can occur when glucose management fails and blood sugar levels become dangerously low or high.

The tissues and cells that make up the human body are living creatures that need sustenance to survive. Glucose is the sort of sugar that cells consume. The body's cells are fully reliant on the bloodstream in which they are bathed to carry glucose to them since they are fixed in place. The body's cells have nothing to fuel themselves with if they don't have enough glucose, and they die quickly.

Food, not glucose, is consumed by humans. As part of the natural digestion process, human meals are turned into glucose. Glucose enters the bloodstream after being converted, causing the level of dissolved glucose in the blood to rise. The dissolved glucose is subsequently carried by the bloodstream to the body's numerous tissues and cells.

Even though glucose is present in the blood, adjacent cells cannot access it without the help of a chemical hormone called insulin. Insulin works like a key to unlock the cells, allowing them to take in and use glucose. In the presence of insulin, cells absorb glucose from the blood, lowering blood sugar levels as sugar leaves the circulation and enters the cells. Insulin functions as a glucose bridge between the bloodstream and the cells. It's critical to realize that as insulin levels rise, blood sugar levels fall (because the sugar goes into the cells to be used for energy).

The body is designed to regulate and buffer the quantity of glucose dissolved in the blood in order to keep a constant supply of glucose to meet cell needs. One of your body's major organs, the pancreas, creates, stores, and releases insulin into the bloodstream to lower glucose levels.

The number and type of meals people consume determine the amount of glucose accessible in their bloodstream at any given time. Glucose is easily broken down from refined carbohydrates, candy, and sweets. As a result, blood glucose levels rise quickly after eating these items. After eating more complex, unprocessed carbs (oatmeal, apples, baked potatoes, etc.) that require more digestive stages before glucose can be given, blood sugars climb steadily and slowly. When blood glucose levels rise quickly, the body must react swiftly by releasing huge amounts of insulin all at once or it risks developing a severe condition known as hyperglycemia (high blood sugar), which will be discussed further below.

Insulin allows cells to use glucose, and glucose concentrations fall as a result. While glucose levels fluctuate quickly, insulin levels fluctuate considerably more slowly. When a lot of simple sugar is consumed, the bloodstream becomes quickly overwhelmed with glucose. In reaction to the increased sugar, the pancreas releases insulin. The glucose enters the cells quickly, but the elevated insulin levels linger in the bloodstream for a long time. This can lead to an excess of insulin in the blood, which can cause hunger and even hypoglycemia (low blood sugar), which is a dangerous condition. There is less of a need for drastic adjustment when blood glucose levels rise gradually. Insulin can be released in a more controlled and safe manner, putting less burden on the body. For a longer amount of time, this slower process will make you feel "full" or content. For these reasons, it is important to restrict the amount and frequency of sweets and refined sugars in your diet for overall health. Consume more complex sugars like raw fruit, whole wheat bread and pasta, and beans instead. The contrast between white (simple) and whole wheat (more complex) bread exemplifies the difference between simple and complex sugars (carbohydrates).

Insulin is essential for a cell's ability to utilize glucose. Problems with insulin production or how the cells sense insulin can quickly throw the body's finely calibrated glucose metabolism system out of whack. Diabetes develops when either of these conditions occurs, blood sugar levels rise and fall, and the body is at risk of being injured.

Symptoms of Diabetes Mellitus

The symptoms of diabetes are brought on by a rise in blood sugar.

Symptoms in general

The following are some of the most common diabetic symptoms:

- More Hunger
- Weight loss due to increased thirst
- Hazy vision due to frequent urine
- Extreme exhaustion
- Wounds that heal slowly or never heal

Men's Symptoms

Men with diabetes may experience diminished sex drive, erectile dysfunction (ED), and inadequate physical strength, in addition to the normal symptoms of diabetes.

Women's Symptoms

Urinary tract infections, yeast infections, and dry, itchy skin are all signs of diabetes in women.

Because most women need to urinate more frequently and feel hungrier during pregnancy, these symptoms aren't usually indicative of diabetes. However, it is critical to have your blood sugar checked because excessive blood sugar can cause difficulties for both you and your baby.

Causes of Diabetes Mellitus

Diabetes can be caused by a variety of factors, including your genetic makeup, family history, ethnicity, health, and environment. Because the causes of diabetes vary based on the individual and the type, there is no one-size-fits-all diabetes cause.

Genetic factors

Scientists have previously postulated the "thrifty gene" as a possible explanation for Black Americans' higher diabetes prevalence. Previous populations assumed to have been subjected to periods of famine were more likely to retain fat efficiently, especially in times of abundance, according to this notion.

According to this theory, an increase in overall body weight, and consequently an increase in diabetes, would occur in modern America.

However, because African Americans are such a diverse group, especially genetically, this theory may not always hold water. Another theory proposes that a higher prevalence of G6PD deficiency in Black guys, combined with a normal "Western diet," may increase diabetes risk.

Health factors

Obesity is one of the most important risk factors for Type 2 diabetes development. Obesity rates are higher among black Americans, particularly among black women than among white Americans. Black Americans endure disadvantages such as poorer socioeconomic position and limited access to nutritional food, which could contribute to the greater obesity rates.

Diabetes risk is considerably raised when poor physical activity levels are combined, especially in Black women and adolescent girls.

Insulin resistance appears to be more common in Black Americans, particularly in Black teens. Insulin resistance has been linked to the development of Type 2 diabetes, which could explain the higher risk of developing the disease. Even so, no single risk factor for diabetes exists, including among African-Americans.

Social factors

Healthcare results and the chance of having certain health disorders are influenced by socioeconomic variables.

Diabetes rates are greater among Black Americans and poor white Americans than among non-poor white Americans.

Furthermore, stress levels are higher among under-resourced socioeconomic groups, which is thought to raise diabetes risk in persons who are susceptible to the condition. Several researchers have discovered links between acute and long-term stress and the development of diabetes.

There are a few other factors that could lead to diabetes. The following are some of them:

Diabetes can be caused by **pancreatitis or pancreatectomy**. Pancreatitis, as well as a pancreatectomy, are known to raise the risk of diabetes.

Polycystic Ovary Syndrome (PCOS)

PCOS is a kind of polycystic ova. Obesity-related insulin resistance is one of the fundamental causes of PCOS, and it may also increase the risk of pre-diabetes and Type 2 diabetes.

Cushing's Syndrome

Cushing syndrome is a condition that affects the adrenal glands. This syndrome causes an increase in cortisol production, which leads to higher blood glucose levels. Diabetes can be caused by an excess of cortisol.

Glucagonoma

Patients with glucagonoma may develop diabetes as a result of a lack of equilibrium between insulin and glucagon production levels.

Steroid Diabetes

Glucocorticoid diabetes is a rare kind of diabetes caused by long-term usage of glucocorticoids.

How do you know if you have diabetes?

Regular checkups are one of the most effective methods to avoid Type 2 diabetes. Several tests can be used by your healthcare provider at these checks to check your blood sugar levels and determine your risk of acquiring diabetes.

After an 8 to 12 hour fast, a fasting blood glucose test measures your blood sugar levels, with the following results:

An oral glucose tolerance test monitors your blood sugar levels for two hours after consuming a sugary beverage, with the following results:

An A1C test evaluates your average blood sugar levels over the previous two to three months, and the findings show: If your blood sugar levels are in the prediabetes range, your doctor will most likely advise you to make certain lifestyle modifications to lower your risk of diabetes.

Chapter 2: Types of Diabetes Mellitus

Diabetes is a term that refers to a group of diseases that affect the body's capacity to metabolize glucose, release insulin, or both.

You require the hormone insulin to absorb glucose (sugar) from the meals you eat. Insulin is produced in your pancreas by beta cells. When insulin reaches your body's cells, it binds to receptors that help the cells recognize and absorb glucose from the bloodstream.

We often use the term Diabetes to refer to Diabetes Mellitus but not many people know that it has two main types:

Type 1 Diabetes

Type 2 Diabetes

Let's take a look at these types of diabetes in detail:

Type 1 Diabetes

Type 1 diabetes is a disorder in which your immune system attacks the cells in your pancreas that produce insulin. These are referred to as beta cells. Because the disorder is most commonly diagnosed in adolescents and teenagers, it was previously known as "juvenile diabetes".

Secondary diabetes is similar to Type 1, but your beta cells are destroyed by something other than your immune systems, such as a disease or an injury to your pancreas.

Both of these conditions are distinct from Type 2 diabetes, which occurs when your body does not respond to insulin as it should.

Symptoms of Type 1 Diabetes

The signs can be modest at first, but they can quickly escalate. They are as follows:

> Increased hunger as a result of extreme thirst (especially after eating)

> Mouth is parched

> Vomiting and an upset stomach

> Urination on a regular basis

> Weight loss that is unexplained even though you are eating and feeling hungry

> Fatigue

> Vision gets compromised (blurry)

> Breathing that is heavy and laborious (your doctor may call this Kussmaul respiration)

> Infections involving the skin, urinary tract, or vaginal area

> Irritability or mood swings

> Bedwetting is a youngster who has previously stayed dry at night

The following are symptoms of Type 1 diabetic emergency:

> Uncertainty and tremors

> Breathing quickly

> Your breath has a fruity scent to it

> Pain in the stomach

> Consciousness loss (rare)

Consequences of Type 1 Diabetes

Insulin is a hormone that aids in the transport of sugar (glucose) into the body's tissues. It is used as a source of energy by your cells.

The process is thrown off when beta cells are damaged due to Type 1 diabetes. Because insulin isn't present, glucose isn't able to enter your cells. Instead, it accumulates in your blood, starving your cells. This raises blood sugar levels, which might result in dehydration. You pee more when you have too much sugar in your blood. That is your body's method of eliminating it. The urine excretes a considerable volume of water, leading your body to become dehydrated.

Loss of Weight

When you pee, glucose leaves your body and takes calories with it. That's why a lot of people with diabetes lose weight. Dehydration is also a factor.

Diabetic Ketoacidosis (DKA)

When your body runs out of glucose, it turns to fat cells for energy. Ketones are produced as a result of this process. To assist you, your liver releases the sugar it has stored. However, without insulin, your body can't utilize it, so it builds up in your blood, along with the acidic ketones. Ketoacidosis is a life-threatening condition caused by a combination of excess glucose, dehydration, and acid accumulation.

Your body will be harmed

High blood glucose levels can injure the neurons and small blood vessels in your eyes, kidneys, and heart over time. They can also increase your risk of atherosclerosis, or hardening of the arteries, which can lead to heart attacks and strokes.

Type 1 diabetes cannot be prevented. Doctors are unsure of all the factors that contribute to it. They are aware, however, that your genes have a role.

They also understand that you can develop Type 1 diabetes if something in your environment, such as a virus, triggers your immune system to attack your pancreas. Autoantibodies, which are present in the majority of persons with Type 1 diabetes, are symptoms of an infection. They're present in practically everyone with diabetes who has a high blood sugar level.

Other autoimmune disorders, such as Graves' disease or vitiligo, can coexist with Type 1 diabetes.

Risk Factors of Type 1 Diabetes

Type 1 diabetes affects just approximately 5% of diabetics. It affects both men and women equally. If you have any of the following, you're more likely to contract it:

> Are you under the age of 20 and white?

> Do you have a Type 1 parent or sibling?

Diagnosis of Type 1 Diabetes

Your blood sugar levels will be checked if your doctor suspects you have Type 1 diabetes. They may test your urine for glucose or substances produced by your body when you are insulin deficient.

Causes of Type 1 Diabetes

Type 1 diabetes has a number of causes.

Type 1 diabetes has an unknown etiology. What is known is that your immune system, which is generally responsible for fighting harmful bacteria and viruses, assaults and destroys your pancreas' insulin-producing cells. You will have very little or no insulin as a result. Sugar builds up in your bloodstream instead of being delivered to your cells.

Type 1 diabetes is assumed to be caused by a mix of genetic predisposition and environmental factors. However, the exact nature of those variables is unknown. Weight isn't thought to play a role in Type 1 diabetes.

Type 2 Diabetes

Type 2 diabetes is a chronic illness that prevents your body from properly utilizing insulin. Insulin resistance is a term used to describe the condition of people with Type 2 diabetes. This type of diabetes is more common in people in their forties and fifties. It was previously known as "adult-onset diabetes". However, Type 2 diabetes also affects children and teenagers, owing to childhood obesity.

Type 2 diabetes is the most frequent type. Type 2 diabetes affects around 29 million people in the United States. Another 84 million people have prediabetes, which means their blood sugar (or blood glucose) is high but not yet high enough to be classified as diabetes.

Signs and Symptoms of Type 2 Diabetes

Type 2 diabetes symptoms might be so subtle that they remain unnoticed. It affects around 8 million people who are unaware of it. Among the signs and symptoms are as follows:

> Being extremely thirsty

> A lot of peeing

> Vision is blurry

> Being irritable

> Numbness or tingling in your hands or feet

> Fatigue or a sense of exhaustion

> Wounds that refuse to heal

> Yeast infections that don't go away

> Feeling hungry

> Weight loss without exerting effort

> Developing new infections

Consult your doctor if you experience dark rashes around your neck or armpits. These are known as acanthosis nigricans and can indicate that your body is becoming insulin resistant.

Causes of Type 2 Diabetes

Insulin is a hormone produced by your pancreas. It aids in the conversion of glucose, a form of sugar, from the food you eat into energy in your cells. Type 2 diabetics produce insulin, but their cells don't use it as well as they should.

To get glucose into your cells, your pancreas produces more insulin initially. However, it finally becomes unable to keep up, and glucose builds up in your bloodstream. Type 2 diabetes is usually caused by a combination of factors. Genes could be one of them. Different pieces of DNA that control how your body generates insulin have been discovered by scientists.

Insulin resistance can be caused by being overweight or obese, especially if you carry your additional pounds around your midsection. The fatty cells surround the healthy cells of the body and hence insulin cannot enter the cell to be utilized.

Metabolic syndrome is a condition in which the body's metabolism is disrupted. Insulin resistance is associated with a slew of symptoms, including high blood sugar, belly fat, high blood pressure, and high cholesterol and triglycerides.

Your liver is producing too much glucose. When your blood sugar falls below a certain level, your liver produces and releases glucose. Your blood sugar rises after you eat, and your liver generally slows down and stores the glucose for later. Some people's livers, however, do not. They continue to produce sugar.

Cellular communication is poor. Cells can send incorrect signals or do not receive messages correctly. A chain reaction can result in diabetes if these issues alter how your cells create and utilize insulin or glucose.

Beta cells that have been broken can cause this condition, too. Your blood sugar is thrown off if the cells that generate insulin send out the wrong quantity of insulin at the wrong time. High blood sugar levels can also harm these cells.

Your cells become resistant to the action of insulin in prediabetes which can develop into Type 2 diabetes, and your pancreas is unable to create enough insulin to overcome this resistance. Sugar accumulates up in your bloodstream instead of going into your cells, where it is needed for energy.

It's unclear why this happens, while genetic and environmental variables are thought to play a role in the development of Type 2 diabetes. Although being overweight is significantly connected to the development of Type 2 diabetes, not everyone who has the disease is obese.

Risk Factors for Type 2 Diabetes

Certain factors increase your chances of developing Type 2 diabetes. The more of them that apply to you, the more likely you are to obtain them. Some items are linked to your identity:

> 45 years old or older

> Family: A diabetic parent, sister, or brother

> Ethnicity: Asian American, African American, Alaska Native, Native American, Hispanic or Latino, or Pacific Islander American

The following are some of the risk factors related to your health and medical history:

> Prediabetes

> Diseases of the heart and blood vessels

> Even if it's treated and under control, high blood pressure can be dangerous.

> HDL ("good") cholesterol levels are low.

> Triglyceride levels are high.

> Obesity or being overweight

> Having a baby that weighed more than 9 pounds

> While you were pregnant, you developed gestational diabetes.

> Polycystic ovarian syndrome (PCOS) is a type of polycystic ova (PCOS)

> Depression

Other factors that increase your diabetes risk include your daily behaviors and lifestyle. These are the ones over which you have control:

> Exercising infrequently or not at all

> Smoking

> Stress

> Too little or too much sleep

Diagnosis and Tests of Type 2 Diabetes

Your blood can be tested for indicators of Type 2 diabetes by your doctor. They'll usually test you again in two days to confirm the diagnosis. However, if your blood glucose is extremely high or you have numerous symptoms, one test may be sufficient.

HBA1c

It's similar to taking an average of your blood glucose levels over the previous two or three months.

Plasma glucose levels after a fast

A high fasting blood sugar test is also known as diabetes. On an empty stomach, it measures your blood sugar. For the 8 hours leading up to the test, you won't be able to eat or drink anything except water.

Oral glucose tolerance test (OGTT)

This test measures your blood glucose levels before and after you consume anything sweet to evaluate how your body reacts to sugar.

Preventing Type 2 Diabetes

Adopting a healthy lifestyle can help you reduce your diabetes risk.

Reduce your weight*:* By losing just 7% to 10% of your body weight, you can lower your risk of Type 2 diabetes in half.

Get moving*:* A daily stroll of thirty minutes at a brisk pace reduces your risk by about a third.

Eat healthily*:* High-processed carbohydrates, sugary drinks, and trans and saturated fats should all be avoided. Limit your intake of red and processed meats.

Stop smoking*:* Consult your doctor about how to avoid gaining weight after you quit smoking, so you don't cause yourself more problems.

> Take your diabetes drugs or insulin as prescribed on a regular basis.

> Examine your blood sugar levels.

> Eat a balanced diet and don't skip meals.

> Check in with your doctor frequently to look for early indicators of concern.

Form a Health-Care Team
Many medical professionals can assist you in living a healthy life with diabetes, including:

> Endocrinologists

> Nurses

> Dietitians with a license to practice

> Pharmacists

> Educators on diabetes

> Doctors of Podiatry

> ophthalmologists

> Dentists

Chapter 3: Reversal of Diabetes Type 1

So, we have learned from the previous chapter that Type 1 diabetes is not caused by a person's dietary habits or lifestyle. It is an autoimmune disease in which the body's immune system targets and destroys healthy pancreatic cells by mistake. While Type 1 diabetes is most commonly diagnosed in children and young adults, it can develop at any age.

Can Diabetes Type 1 Be TURNED AROUND?

When a person is diagnosed with Type 1 diabetes, one of the first questions they ask is, "Is there a therapy?" The answer is, unfortunately, "NO". While Type 1 diabetes may be controlled or managed with insulin, a healthy diet, and exercise, there is presently no therapy. Researchers at the Diabetes Research Institute, on the other hand, are currently working on ways to turn around the illness, so that patients with Type 1 diabetes can live healthy lives without the use of medication.

For almost a century, therapy for Type 1 diabetes has focused on disease management. Patients may now regulate their blood glucose levels with frequent insulin injections or an insulin pump thanks to medical advances in the past.

Treatments are being researched to medicate Type 1 diabetes and restore the body's natural ability to produce insulin. Some patients are already living insulin-free as a result of these studies, which has improved significantly their quality of life.

Biological Therapy

Type 1 diabetes is more difficult to prevent, although similar lifestyle modifications can help to delay the onset and severity of the illness. But researchers are finding some biological therapies to turn around diabetes.

Islet Cell Transplantation

A biological therapy is a treatment that enables the body to produce insulin again, bringing blood sugar levels to normal levels without further complications.

This study focuses on a method known as "islet transplantation". Islets are pancreatic cell clusters that work together to control blood sugar. In an islet transplant, surgeons extract healthy islets from an organ donor's pancreas and inject them into a patient with Type 1 diabetes. In studies, some individuals who have undergone this process were able to minimize or eliminate their need for insulin injections.

Steps

Dietary Reference Intakes (DRI) studies have extensively demonstrated that islet transplantation can eliminate the requirement for insulin injections. They are currently working on further research so that more individuals can benefit from this treatment.

The three primary study topics of the BioHub, known commonly as the "Three S's" — **Site, Sustain, and Supply** — are being pursued concurrently by DRI's varied team of scientists, in coordination with a global network of collaborators.

Site

Donor islets have traditionally been transplanted into the liver, although this implant site has several limits, leading DRI experts to look for alternate options. Researchers are now working on developing a mini-endocrine pancreas at a location within the body that can house transplanted islets, as well as other "helper" technologies that preserve the cells without the usage of anti-rejection medicines.

Sustain

Several strategies are being studied by researchers to ensure the long-term survival of the islets. Some strategies use protective barriers to safeguard cells, while others include providing oxygen or other helpful substances to the transplant environment. Ultimately, maintaining the cells' survival is about interfering with the autoimmune response that caused Type 1Diabetes to develop.

Supply

Currently, islet cells used for transplantation come from donor pancreases, but there are not enough organs to treat the millions of children and adults living with diabetes. DRI researchers are developing ways to create a reliable and plentiful supply of insulin-producing cells, or even regenerate a patient's pancreatic cells.

One problem that lies within this treatment is "organ rejection". The same autoimmune reaction that attacked the recipient's original islet cells might destroy the transplanted islet cells. Furthermore, like with other organ transplants, the recipient must take immunosuppressive medicines to prevent the body from rejecting the transplanted islet cells.

If the body can suppress autoimmunity, it may be able to restore a person's insulin-producing cells, resulting in a natural supply within the body.

Progress

According to recent research conducted by DRI experts, a small group of patients who had islet transplants was able to live without insulin injections for ten years while maintaining blood sugar levels in the same range as persons who had never received insulin injections.

Within the recent year, also advancements in islet transplantation have been made: Islets that are encapsulated in microcapsules are less likely to be attacked by the body's immune system.

Limitation

Although islet transplants have the potential to be generally beneficial in the treatment of Type 1 diabetes, and their limitations are being addressed by current research, they are still not suitable for all Type 1 diabetics. This applies especially to those who require extra amounts of insulin every day or those who are overweight. Besides, a limitation of donors prevents this type of treatment from positively impacting as many Type 1 diabetics as it could.

Gene Therapy

Because Type 1 diabetes is a genetic disease, a genetic treatment may hold the key to a true solution. Gene therapy is a method of treatment in which specific genes that cause disease are targeted and then altered. This can either prevent the disease from developing or medicate the condition caused by the disease. At the moment, gene therapies have only been used to treat a few rare disorders.

Immunotherapy

Treating the immune system in Type 1 diabetes is a significant area of active study. Remember that Type 1 diabetes is a condition in which the body's immune system assaults the pancreas. Immunotherapy is the use of drugs that attempt to disable components of the immune system that are involved in Type 1 diabetes. Human clinical studies of these pharmaceuticals are already ongoing, but keep in mind that, similarly to a pancreas transplant, this form of treatment may relieve you of the need for insulin, but you will still need to take some regular medication to maintain and reach the effectiveness of procedure you went through.

Managing Diabetes Type 1 Along With Insulin

Sometimes the question arises of why we need to manage our diabetes Type 1 when we have to take insulin. The answer is diet and physical exercise are important in the treatment of Type 1 diabetes' ABCs (A1C, Blood pressure, and Cholesterol). It is essential to understand how to balance dietary choices, physical activity, and insulin to effectively manage glycated hemoglobin (A1C) and establish stable blood sugar levels.

Treatment for Type 1 Diabetes

Type 1 diabetes patients can live long and healthy lives. You'll need to monitor your blood sugar levels closely. Your doctor will tell you a range of numbers that you should stick to. As needed, make adjustments to your insulin, food, and activities. Insulin shots are required for all people with Type 1 diabetes who want to keep their blood sugar under control.

When your doctor talks about insulin, three topics will come up:

- The time it takes for the medication to reach your system and start decreasing your blood sugar is referred to as "onset."
- Insulin is most effective in decreasing blood sugar during "peak time."
- "Duration" refers to how long it works after it starts.
- Insulin comes in a variety of forms.
- In about 15 minutes, rapid-acting medication begins to work. It works for 2 to 4 hours after you take it, peaking around 1 hour after you take it.
- Regular or short-acting medication takes roughly 30 minutes to start working. It reaches its peak between 2 and 3 hours and continues to work for 3 to 6 hours.
- Intermediate-acting medications take 2 to 4 hours to reach your bloodstream after injection. It works for 12 to 18 hours and peaks between 4 and 12 hours.
- Long-acting medication takes many hours to enter your system and lasts for around 24 hours.
- Your doctor may begin by injecting you with two types of insulin twice a day. You could need extra shots later.

The majority of insulin comes in a vial, which is a little glass bottle. You use a syringe with a needle on the end to draw it out and give yourself the shot. Some types have a pre-filled pen. A third type is inhaled. You can also obtain it from a pump, which is a device that you wear, and inject it into your body via a little tube. Your doctor will assist you in determining the optimal type and delivery technique for you.

Lifestyle Changes

The importance of exercise in the treatment of Type 1 diabetes cannot be overstated. It is not, however, as simple as going for a run. Blood sugar levels are affected by exercise. As a result, any exercise, including basic jobs around the house or yard, must be balanced with your insulin dose and the food you eat.

Knowledge is a powerful tool. To see how activity affects you, check your blood sugar before, during, and after it. Some items will cause your levels to rise, while others will not. To protect your insulin from dipping too low, you can increase it or eat a carb-rich snack.

If your blood sugar is above 240 mg/dL, then go for a ketone test. Ketones are the acids that might come from high sugar levels. If they're fine, you're good to go. If they're buzzed, don't do the workout.

You'll also need to know how diet impacts blood sugar levels. You can create a healthy eating plan that helps keep your levels where they should be once you understand the functions that carbs, lipids, and protein play. You can get started with the support of a diabetic educator or a licensed dietician. We have also mentioned dietary guidelines for diabetics. Besides, you will also be given some diabetic recipes in the last chapter.

Making healthy dietary choices daily provides both immediate and long-term benefits. It is possible to eat healthily and control diabetes with education, experience, and guidance from a dietitian and/or a diabetes educator.

Importance of Diet

Many factors influence how effectively diabetes is managed. Many of these factors are all under the control of the diabetic, such as how much and what is eaten, how frequently blood sugar is monitored, physical activity levels, and the accuracy and consistency of medication or insulin doses. Even minor modifications can have an impact on blood sugar control.

Eating a consistent amount of food every day and taking insulin as prescribed can significantly improve blood sugar control and lower the risk of diabetes-related complications such as coronary artery disease, renal disease, and nerve damage. Furthermore, these measures have an impact on weight control. A dietician can assist you in developing a meal plan that is specific to your medical needs, lifestyle, and personal preferences. Otherwise, you will need to increase the insulin doses more frequently.

Relation between Diabetes Type 1 and Meal Timing

For some people, eating at the same time every day is important, especially for those who take the same dosage of insulin at the same time every day (called a "fixed regimen"). You are at risk of developing low blood glucose if a meal is skipped or delayed.

People requiring extensive insulin therapy (an insulin pump or multiple daily insulin injections) have more meal timing flexibility. Skipping or delaying a meal does not usually raise the risk of low blood sugar with these regimens.

High Fat and High Protein Foods

High-fat, high-protein meals digest slower than low-fat, low-protein ones. High-fat foods and meals can be consumed occasionally. When rapid-acting insulin is being used before a meal, blood sugar levels may drop quickly after eating a high-fat meal and then increase hours later. People who eat more protein or fat than usual may need to increase their insulin dose at mealtime to manage the delayed rise in blood sugar.

Carbohydrates

When calculating carbs, keep the serving size and fiber grams in mind. Eating more than one serving raises the number of calories and carbs taken, as well as the amount of insulin required to cover the meal. Some packaged snacks, for example, contain two or more servings. Multiply the number of servings by the number of carbs to get the total carbohydrate content of the package.

A dietitian can generally help you figure out how many carbs you need at each meal and snack depending on your regular eating patterns, insulin regimen, body weight, nutritional objectives, and level of exercise. The majority of diabetics indicate a moderate carbohydrate consumption (44 to 46 percent of total calories).

General Recommendations

Except for the following recommendations, which are mostly identical to the recommendations for the general population, the American Diabetes Association (ADA) nutritional guidelines do not include specific total dietary compositional recommendations.

1. Carbohydrates from fruits, vegetables, whole grains, legumes, and low-fat milk are recommended. Diabetes patients are recommended to avoid sugar-sweetened drinks (including fruit juice).
2. The ideal carbohydrate intake is unknown. Monitoring carbohydrate intake (basic or advanced carbohydrate counting) is important in diabetic patients because carbohydrate intake directly determines postprandial blood sugar, and appropriate insulin adjustment for identified carbohydrate quantities is one of the most important factors that can improve glycemic control.
3. Meals with a low glycemic index and glycemic load, in addition to total carbs, may give a minor additional benefit for glycemic control.
4. Several dietary practices are allowed (low fat, low carbohydrate, Mediterranean, vegetarian).
5. The quality of fat is more significant than the quantity of fat. Saturated and trans fats are risk factors for coronary heart disease (CHD), but monounsaturated and polyunsaturated fats are beneficial. Diabetes puts people at a higher risk for heart disease and stroke and eating a diet low in saturated fat, trans fats, and cholesterol can help lower cholesterol levels and reduce these risks.
6. Saturated fats (found in meat, cheese, and ice cream, for example) can

be substituted with monounsaturated and polyunsaturated fatty acids (for example in fish, olive oil, nuts). Trans fatty acid intake should be kept to a minimum. Trans fats are no longer permitted in processed foods in the United States. Although relatively minute levels of trans fats are naturally present in meat, poultry, and dairy products, the amount is negligible to be concerned about.

Avoiding Weight Gain in Diabetes

Weight gain is a potential adverse effect of Type 1 diabetes intensive insulin treatment. The following tips are advised to avoid weight gain.

a. Measuring your weight regularly is essential (once weekly). Weight gain of more than 2 to 3 pounds indicates that you should reduce your calorie intake or increase your physical activity.
b. To avoid weight gain, you may need to reduce your calorie intake by 250 to 300 calories as your blood sugar control improves.
c. If your blood sugar levels are consistently low at a certain time of day, talk to your doctor about reducing your insulin dose rather than adding a snack.

Exercise

a. Regular exercise can help you lose weight and keep it off. Most days of the week, 30 minutes of exercise daily is advised.
b. Insulin-dependent people should monitor their blood sugar levels before and after exercise. If you exercise intensely and for an extended period (more than thirty minutes), check your blood sugar every 15 minutes (if the exercise regimen is new and supposed to be repeated). Monitoring your blood sugar levels regularly can help you gain a sense of how exercise affects your blood sugar level.

Chapter 4: Reversal of Diabetes Type 2

Diabetes Type 2 is a severe, long-term medical problem. It mostly affects adults, although it is becoming progressively prevalent in children as the rate of obesity increases across all age groups. Type 2 diabetes is caused by several reasons. The most significant factors include being overweight or obese.

Can You TURN AROUND Diabetes Type 2?

Type 2 diabetes has the potential to be fatal. However, if properly treated, it can be managed or even turned around. According to recent studies, Type 2 diabetes cannot be medicated, although patients can have glucose levels that return to the non-diabetic range (full remission) or pre-diabetes glucose levels (partial remission).

The simplest practice for people with Type 2 diabetes to achieve remissions is to reduce a significant amount of weight. We talk about remission instead of therapy because it isn't permanent. The beta cells have been impaired, but the underlying genetic variables that contribute to the person's susceptibility to diabetes are not altered. Although remission can be achieved by regular medical treatments like lifestyle changes, many remissions are the result of gastric bypass surgery. These individuals frequently have a complete or partial reversal of high glucose levels. Even before considerable weight-reduction occurs, the surgery's change in hormonal balance leads to improved glucose metabolism.

Treatment for Reversing or Managing Diabetes Type 2

Although Type 2 diabetes is a significant health issue, it is treatable. You can manage Type 2 diabetes, keep blood sugar levels under control, avoid complications, and stay healthy and active for many years with therapy and lifestyle modifications. Your healthcare practitioner may use a variety of tests to manage Type 2 diabetes. Type 2 diabetes is treated with a combination of lifestyle changes and medication.

Changes in your way of life

You might be able to achieve your goal blood sugar levels only with food and exercise.

Loss of weight

Getting rid of excess weight can help. While decreasing 5% of your body weight is beneficial, losing at least 7% and maintaining it appears to be optimum. That indicates that just decreasing roughly 13 pounds, someone who weighs 180 pounds can change their blood sugar levels. Weight loss can seem daunting, but starting with portion management and eating healthy foods is an excellent place to start.

Eating well is important

Type 2 diabetes does not require a special diet. A licensed dietician can educate you on carbs and assist you in developing a meal plan that you can stick to. Concentrate on:

> Lowering your calorie intake

> Reducing refined carbohydrates, particularly sweets

> Including more fruits and vegetables in your diet

> Increasing your fiber intake

Exercise

Every day, try to get 30 to 60 minutes of physical activity. You can exercise by walking, biking, swimming, or doing anything else that raises your heart rate. Combine this with a strength-training program, such as yoga or weightlifting. You might need a snack before an exercise if you're on a blood sugar-lowering prescription.

Keep an eye on your blood sugar levels

Your doctor will tell you whether or not you need to test your blood sugar levels and how often you should do so, depending on your therapy, especially if you're on insulin.

Medication

If lifestyle changes aren't enough to get you to your goal blood sugar levels, medication may be required. Metformin is one of the most commonly prescribed medications for Type 2 diabetes (Fortamet, Glucophage, Glumetza, Riomet). When it comes to Type 2 diabetes, this is usually the first prescription prescribed. It helps your body respond better to the insulin it does make by lowering the quantity of glucose your liver produces.

Sulfonylureas

This class of medications aids in the production of insulin in the body. Glimepiride (Amaryl), glipizide (Glucotrol, Metaglip), and glyburide are some of them (DiaBeta, Micronase).

Meglitinides

They aid in the production of insulin and are more effective than sulfonylureas. Nateglinide (Starlix) or repaglinide are two options (Prandin).

Thiazolidinediones

They, like metformin, increase insulin sensitivity. Pioglitazone (Actos) or rosiglitazone (Rosiglitazone) are two options (Avandia). However, because they increase your risk of cardiac problems, they aren't normally the initial therapeutic option.

Inhibitors of DPP-4

These drugs — linagliptin (Tradjenta), saxagliptin (Onglyza), and sitagliptin (Januvia) — reduce blood sugar levels but can potentially cause joint discomfort and pancreas inflammation.

Agonists for the GLP-1 receptor

These drugs are administered through a needle to slow digestion and lower blood sugar levels. Exenatide (Byetta, Bydureon), liraglutide (Victoza), and semaglutide (Ozempic) are three of the most frequent drugs.

Inhibitors of SGLT2

These aid in the filtering of more glucose by your kidneys. You could be prescribed canagliflozin (Invokana), dapagliflozin (Farxiga), or empagliflozin (Empagliflozin, Jardiance). Empagliflozin has also been shown to reduce the risk of heart failure-related hospitalization or mortality.

Insulin

Long-acting insulins, such as insulin detemir (Levemir) or insulin glargine, may be used at night (Lantus).

Even if you make lifestyle changes and take your medication as prescribed, your blood sugar levels may worsen with time. This does not mean you have made a mistake. Diabetes is a gradual disease, and many people will eventually require many medications.

Combination therapy is when you take more than one drug to control your Type 2 diabetes.

You and your doctor should collaborate to choose the optimum combination for you. Typically, you'll continue to take metformin while adding something else.

What that is may vary depending on your circumstances. Some medicines, for example, decrease blood sugar rises (which your doctor may refer to as hyperglycemia) that occur shortly after meals. Others are better at preventing blood sugar decreases (hypoglycemia) between meals. Some may aid in weight loss, cholesterol reduction, and diabetic management.

Any probable adverse effects should be discussed with your doctor. The cost could also be a concern.

If you are on medication for something else, you will need to consider that while making a selection.

When you start taking a new drug combination, you will need to see your doctor more frequently.

It's possible that adding a second drug won't help you control your blood sugar. Alternatively, the combination of two medications may only be effective for a brief period. If this should be the case, your doctor may suggest a third noninsulin medicine, or you may need to begin insulin therapy.

To medicate diabetes, you must be sufficient to inhibit the cycle by taking breaks on your insulin-producing cells. Type 2 treatments include:

Low-Calories Diet

A low-calorie, low-carbohydrate diet is important for lowering the amount of insulin the body needs to produce, resulting in less insulin resistance. This may include eating more fresh fruits and vegetables, whole grains, and other high-fiber, nutritious meals; avoiding sugary beverages, processed foods, sweets, and refined carbohydrates; and substituting saturated fats with healthy fats such as olive oil. It's also essential to take frequent meals and snacks to keep blood sugar levels consistent. To maintain a healthy weight, you may also need to eat smaller portion sizes and consume fewer calories.

Physical Activity

Physical activity can help manage blood sugar levels. Therefore, exercise is an important element of controlling Type 2 diabetes. At the same time, sitting for extended periods can worsen your diabetes. Therefore, it's important to walk around. Aim for 30 minutes of aerobic activity every day, such as walking, jogging, dancing, or cycling, plus two or three sessions of strength training or other resistance activities, such as weight lifting, on most days of the week.

Before starting an exercise program, consult with your doctor to ensure that it is safe for your health problems.

Weight loss

If you are overweight, losing some of that may be beneficial to your health. Even reducing 5% of your body weight can enhance your body's capacity to control blood sugar, blood pressure, cholesterol, and triglycerides. As you lose weight, your body's insulin reduces your blood sugar levels more efficiently, causing your A1c readings (glycated hemoglobin) to decline over time. In one study, persons with Type 2 diabetes who shed 5% to 10% of their body weight were 3 times more likely to drop their A1c (glycated hemoglobin) by 0.5 percent. You may have a different weight-loss goal in mind, or you may be considering other health issues. The advantages increase with greater weight reduction. It's important to lose weight at a healthy rate, so consult with your healthcare team to develop a weight loss regimen.

Blood Sugar Monitoring

People with Type 2 Diabetes may constantly check their blood sugar levels to ensure they are not either high or too low. Most individuals do this at home using a blood glucose meter, which takes a drop of blood and measures the amount of sugar in it. You should check your blood sugar levels once or twice a day, or before exercising.

Medication

Several medications may be prescribed by your doctor to help your body use insulin more efficiently and keep blood sugars under control. It may help in the treatment of other diabetes-related health issues such as hypertension and cardiovascular disease. Through diet and exercise, you can reliably reduce your A1c (glycated hemoglobin). However, if your doctor has recommended medicine, such as **metformin, miglitol, or insulin,**

- Sulfonylureas and glinides, both of which can increase insulin production.
- Thiazolidinediones, which can boost insulin sensitivity.
- DPP-4 inhibitors and GLP-1 receptor agonists help reduce blood glucose levels.
- SGLT2 inhibitors can help the body in excreting excess glucose in the urine.

you must take medication as directed. If you frequently skip doses, your blood sugar levels may rise, causing your A1c (glycated hemoglobin) to rise. However, if you adhere to your doctor's medication regime and follow all of your sessions, your blood sugar should stay under control, and your A1c will reflect that. Tell your doctor that you want to work on reducing, or possibly eliminating your medicines. But don't try to stop them on your own.

Insulin Replacement Therapy

While insulin treatment is most commonly linked with Type 1 diabetes, it is also prescribed in Type 2 diabetes patients. Your doctor may prescribe insulin treatment to keep your blood sugar levels constant if your body stops producing insulin or generates inadequate amounts. You may need to increase or change your blood glucose monitoring to determine how much or what type of insulin you require each day to control your glucose levels.

Alternative Medication Or Therapies

Many patients find that alternative treatments can supplement their Type 2 diabetes therapy and reduce some of the symptoms of the disease. Acupuncture, acupressure, and massage are all therapies that can assist with relaxation, circulation, and nerve pain. Although stress can lead to complications such as high blood pressure, many people with Type 2 diabetes find meditation or mindful breathing to be beneficial. Yoga and tai chi can also aid with stress management while also encouraging healthy physical exercise.

While certain methods may be beneficial, others may be ineffective, and yet others may be destructive. Some nutritional supplements can be toxic when taken in large doses, or they may induce a drug interaction with one of your prescriptions. So, it's always a good idea to see your doctor before adopting any alternative therapies.

Bariatric Surgery and Diabetes

Obesity is an issue if it is contributing to your diabetes or making it difficult to regulate your blood sugar levels. By physically reducing the quantity of food you can eat, these procedures can help you shed a considerable amount of weight. Weight reduction surgery is a helpful technique for many people to support and enforce lifestyle changes that will enhance their health and quality of life.

Bariatric surgery isn't just about trying to lose weight for those with diabetes. It is currently considered an effective treatment for Type 2 diabetes, with weight loss as an extra benefit. It improves your body in producing and using insulin more efficiently and effectively

Bariatric surgery alters the digestive system's function. Studies have shown that people's blood sugar levels drop below the diabetic range immediately after surgery, even if they haven't lost weight. As a result, most individuals who have bariatric surgery have their diabetic prescriptions discontinued shortly afterward.

According to one research, over a third (30.4 percent) of persons who underwent surgery remained in remission after 15 years., in ways that benefit people with

Type 2 diabetes. It can help you feel full sooner, which means you eat less. It also can...

a. change the way your gut hormones act, which in turn can influence how your body produces insulin.
b. increase your body's production of bile acids, which makes your body more sensitive to insulin.
c. optimize your body's utilization of insulin, resulting in lower blood sugar levels.

Types Of Bariatric Surgery

1. There are several surgical methods available, such as a gastric band, gastric bypass, or sleeve gastrectomy.
2. Gastric band — a band is wrapped around the upper part of the stomach, which means you won't need to eat as much to feel satisfied.
3. Gastric bypass – the digestive system is rerouted to bypass the majority of the stomach excluding a tiny pouch at the top. You will feel fuller quicker and consume fewer calories.
4. Sleeve gastrectomy — a segment of your stomach is removed, but your intestines are not rerouted. Again, you won't need to eat as much to be satisfied.

When Bariatric Surgeries Are Recommended

Bariatric surgery is performed on the NHS (National Health Service) for those who meet particular criteria. If you are eligible for NHS treatment, you will be referred to an evaluation to determine if surgery is appropriate for you. The NHS guidelines are largely identical to worldwide clinical guidelines released in 2016 by several significant international diabetes organizations, including Diabetes UK. These recommendations also suggest a lower BMI (Body Mass Index) limit for South Asians with Type 2 diabetes. These include:

1. You have a BMI of 40 or higher, or a BMI between 35 and 40, and you have an obesity-related issue that could improve if you lost weight (such as Type 2 diabetes or high blood pressure).

2. You've tried all available weight-loss measures, such as diet and physical activity, but haven't been able to shed or keep the weight off.
3. You agree to long-term follow-up post-surgery, such as healthy lifestyle modifications and regular check-ups.

Chapter 5: Complications of Type 1 Diabetes

Type 1 diabetes, if not well-controlled, can lead to a variety of complications. The following are some of the complications.

Atherosclerosis

Atherosclerosis is a type of cardiovascular disease. Diabetes increases the risk of blood clots, high blood pressure, and high cholesterol. Chest pain, a heart attack, a stroke, or heart failure are all possible outcomes. Diabetes patients have an excess of sugar in their blood. Blood chemistry may be altered, and blood vessels may narrow as a result. Or, it can harm blood vessels.

Atherosclerosis has the following warning signs:

> Pain in the chest

> Breathing problems

> Heart palpitations

> Weakness or vertigo

> Nausea

> Sweating

Infections of the Skin

Infections caused by bacteria or fungi are more common in diabetics. Blisters or rashes can also be caused by diabetes.

Candida albicans are frequently the cause of fungal infections in diabetics. Itchy rashes with wet, red regions surrounded by tiny blisters and scales can be caused by this yeast-like fungus. Infections in the warm, moist folds of the skin are common.

Bacterial skin infections are also more common in people with diabetes. Bacterial infections in the eyelid glands (sty) or deep beneath the skin are possible (boils and carbuncles). Swollen, hot, red, and painful skin is a sign of infection.

Red, red-brown, or skin-colored rashes are all possible. Although medical treatment is rarely necessary, a topical steroid drug such as hydrocortisone may be beneficial.

Gum Disease

Gum disease is a condition that affects the teeth and gums. Mouth difficulties can be caused by a lack of saliva, excessive plaque, and inadequate blood flow.

When your blood sugar is high due to diabetes, the sugar in your saliva surrounding your teeth and under your gums is higher. This promotes the growth of dangerous bacteria and plaque. Plaque causes gum irritation, which can lead to gum disease, tooth decay, and tooth loss. Gum disease causes bleeding, redness, and swelling of the gums.

Controlling your glucose level may be your best tool for managing dry mouth if you have diabetes. Take your medication as directed and stay away from sugary foods and beverages. Consult your doctor if your dry mouth persists. It may be a side effect of your drug.

Pregnancy and Diabetes

Poor diabetes control during pregnancy raises the risk of birth abnormalities and other pregnancy complications. It can also put the woman's health in jeopardy. Prenatal and postnatal health care can help prevent birth abnormalities and other health issues.

Women with Type 1 diabetes are at risk for premature birth, birth defects, stillbirth, and preeclampsia. You have a good chance of having a normal pregnancy and birth if you are healthy and your diabetes is well controlled when you get pregnant. Diabetes that is not effectively controlled during pregnancy might have long-term consequences for you and your baby.

Because they are already producing an excess of insulin, babies born to diabetic mothers are at a higher risk of suffering low blood sugar or hypoglycemia immediately after delivery and during the first few days of life. Diabetic mothers' infants (IDM) are typically larger than other babies, especially if diabetes is poorly managed. This may make vaginal birth more difficult and raise the risk of nerve damage and other birth trauma. Cesarean births are also more common in diabetic women.

Newborns may have very low blood glucose levels at delivery due to the additional insulin produced by the baby's pancreas, and they are also at a higher risk for respiratory issues. Children and adults who are born with too much insulin are at risk of becoming obese and developing Type 2 diabetes. The most common insulin side effect during pregnancy is low blood sugar (hypoglycemia), which can occur if you skip or delay a meal or inject too much insulin.

Retinopathy

This eye condition affects roughly 80% of persons with Type 1 diabetes who have had it for more than 15 years. No matter how long you've had the disease, it's rare before puberty. Keep your blood sugar, blood pressure, cholesterol, and triglycerides under control to avoid it and preserve your vision.

If left misdiagnosed and untreated, it might result in blindness. Diabetic retinopathy, on the other hand, usually takes several years to progress to the point where it threatens your vision. Diabetes causes elevated blood sugar, which leads to diabetic retinopathy. Too much sugar in your blood can damage your retina, which detects light and sends signals to your brain through a nerve at the back of your eye commonly known as the optic nerve. Diabetes wreaks havoc on the body's blood vessels. Diabetic retinopathy is caused by a breakdown of the blood-retinal barrier (BRB) caused by diabetes, which results in vascular leaking of fluid and circulating proteins into the neural retina.

Fluid extravasation into the neural retina causes aberrant retinal thickness and, in some cases, cystoid edema of the macula. Although retinopathy does not normally occur until five years after a diagnosis of Type 1 diabetes, it may already be present when Type 2 Diabetes is discovered. Retinal degeneration affects 98 percent of people with Type 1 diabetes and 78 percent of people with Type 2 diabetes after 15 years.

Kidney Failure

Nephropathy is a disease that affects about 20% to 30% of patients with Type 1 diabetes. Over time, the chances improve. It's most likely to appear 15 to 25 years after diabetes begins. It can lead to major complications such as renal failure and heart disease.

Diabetes causes damage to the body's tiny blood vessels. When the blood arteries in your kidneys are damaged, your kidneys are unable to adequately clear your blood. Your body will retain more water and salt than it should, leading to weight gain and swelling in your ankles. Protein may be present in your urine.

Within two to five years of being diagnosed with Type I diabetes, almost all patients show some signs of functional alteration in the kidneys. Within 10 to 30 years, roughly 30 to 40 percent of people develop more significant renal disease. The kidneys grow less effective at purifying the blood as the damage progresses. The kidneys can stop working if the damage is severe enough.

Kidney damage is irreversible. Because the kidneys produce urine, the urine may vary when the kidneys fail. How? Dark-colored urine is produced and diabetes may cause you to urinate less frequently or in lower amounts than normal. It's possible that blood is present in your pee.

Consume less sodium and salt. That's a smart approach for diabetics, and it's more crucial for people with chronic kidney disease (CKD). Your kidneys lose the ability to regulate your sodium-water balance over time. Lowering your blood pressure and reducing fluid buildup in your body, both of which are frequent symptoms of kidney disease, can be achieved by consuming less sodium in your diet.

Nerve injury and a lack of blood flow

Damaged nerves and hardened arteries cause a loss of feeling in your feet as well as a lack of blood supply. This increases your risk of damage and makes healing open sores and wounds more difficult. You could lose a limb if this happens. Digestive issues such as nausea, vomiting, and diarrhea can also be caused by nerve injury.

You can take precautions to avoid these issues:

✓ Make every effort to keep your blood sugar in check.

✓ Keep an eye on your blood pressure and cholesterol levels.

✓ Eat healthily and do some exercise.

✓ Quit smoking if you're a smoker.

✓ Make sure your feet and teeth are in good shape.

✓ Have your medical, dental, and eye checks done on a regular basis.

Chapter 6: Complications of Type 2 Diabetes

High blood sugar levels can harm and cause difficulties with your heart and blood vessels over time. You're up to five times more likely to develop heart disease or suffer a stroke if you're overweight. You're also at an increased risk of blood vessel blockage (atherosclerosis) and chest discomfort (angina).

Kidneys

You may need dialysis or a kidney transplant if your kidneys are damaged or you have renal failure. In dialysis patients, glycemic management is critical since poor control is linked to a high rate of morbidity and mortality. The diabetes dialysis diet will keep you healthy by controlling your blood glucose levels and lowering your risk of other diabetes and kidney disease problems. According to research, patients on maintenance dialysis (MD) had a life expectancy of 4.5 years for those aged 60 to 64, which is less than most cancers. Patients with diabetic MD have a 1.3-fold greater mortality risk than those with other types of primary renal impairment.

Sleep Apnea

Sleep apnea is a condition in which your breathing repeatedly stops and resumes while you sleep. If you have diabetes, sleep apnea can make managing your diabetes more challenging. This is due to an increase in carbon dioxide in your blood when your breathing pauses while you sleep. Insulin resistance develops as a result of this, and the body is unable to utilize insulin properly. Obstructive sleep apnea (OSA) affects glucose metabolism, causes insulin resistance, and is linked to Type 2 diabetes development. Obesity is an important modulator of OSA's effect on Type 2 diabetes. Continuous positive airway pressure (CPAP) therapy for sleep apnea not only improves sleep quality but also lowers blood sugar (glucose) levels, lowering the risk of diabetes consequences such as heart and renal illness.

Hearing Loss

Hearing difficulties are more likely in you, although it's unclear why. Diabetes might also harm your ears' nerves. High blood sugar levels in the inner ear can damage small blood vessels and nerves over time. Low blood sugar can affect how nerve signals pass from the inner ear to the brain over time. Hearing loss can result from any sort of nerve injury. Diabetes destroys small blood vessels in the inner ear and the vestibular system, which aids in balance. Hearing and balance signals may have a tougher time getting to your brain if you have diabetes. Diabetes patients are more likely to develop hearing loss.

Brain

High blood sugar levels can harm your brain and increase your chances of Alzheimer's disease. Diabetes has been linked to a number of comorbid problems, including mental illnesses such as depression, anxiety, and cognitive impairment. Other vascular and behavioral issues are linked to this connection, which may be mediated by brain oxidative stress and neuronal death.

Sugar is the brain's primary fuel source. As a result, if your blood sugar is out of whack as a result of diabetes, you can experience cognitive fog.

Reduced concentration, for example, is a symptom of brain fog. Other symptoms are:

- Fluctuations in mood
- Issues with memory
- Blood sugar levels that aren't appropriately maintained - blood sugar that is too high or too low might cause brain fog.

Diabetes and brain fog have various effects on different persons. Some people may simply have slight cognitive difficulties, while others may be unable to function or think clearly.

Brain fog symptoms associated with diabetes can include any of the following:

- fatigue

- dizziness
- confusion
- memory loss
- difficulty problem-solving
- trouble finding the right words
- inability to process information
- inability to concentrate
- feeling as if you're moving in slow motion

Depression

Depressed people are twice as likely to suffer from diabetes. So, you're more likely to develop depression if you have diabetes, whether Type 1 or Type 2. Besides, if you're depressed, you're more likely to get Type 2 diabetes. Diabetes and depression may be managed jointly, which is good news.

Discomfort, sadness, anxiety, and disordered eating are all common mental health disorders in people with Type 1 diabetes. These are, however, all curable conditions. It's critical to pay attention to how you feel about having diabetes or caring for someone who does.

The best approach to avoid these problems is to keep your diabetes under control.

Chapter 7: Meals for Diabetics

A meal plan tells you when, what, and how much to eat to provide the nourishment you need while staying within your goal blood sugar range. A smart meal plan will consider your objectives, preferences, and lifestyle, as well as any medications you're taking. The following points must be considered:

- Include additional non-starchy veggies, such as broccoli, spinach, and green beans in your diet plan.
- Include fewer added sugars and refined grains with less than 2 grams of fiber per serving, such as white bread, rice, and pasta.
- As much as possible, focus on whole foods rather than heavily processed items.

Carbohydrates in your food cause your blood sugar to rise. The amount of time it takes for carbs to boost your blood sugar depends on the food and what you consume with it. Drinking fruit juice, for example, boosts blood sugar faster than eating whole fruit. When you combine carbohydrates with foods that contain protein, fat, or fiber, your blood sugar climbs more slowly.

To avoid high or low blood sugar levels, plan for regular, well-balanced meals. It's a good idea to eat around the same quantity of carbs at each meal. Counting carbohydrates and utilizing the plate approach are two popular methods for making meal planning easier.

Carbohydrate Counting

Keeping note of how many carbs you consume and setting a limit for each meal will help you stay within your goal blood sugar range. Consult your doctor or a qualified dietitian to determine how much carbs you can consume per day and per meal, and then look over the list of typical carb-containing foods and serving sizes.

When it comes to successfully managing diabetes, controlling your carbohydrate intake is crucial. Studies have shown that monitoring carb intake leads to better blood glucose (BG) numbers and may improve your health in other ways, too.

To function effectively, your body requires nutrition. Macronutrients are the nutrients it requires in vast numbers, whereas micronutrients are the nutrients it requires in little amounts.

Carbohydrates, proteins, and fats are the three categories of macronutrients. Carbs provide you with energy and provide fuel for your brain. Protein is essential for the health of your tissues and cells. Fat both protects and gives energy to your important organs.

Carbs have the largest impact on blood sugar levels. Carb counting is a method of ensuring that your body receives enough carbohydrates to fuel your everyday activities without causing your blood sugar to rise to harmful levels.

Monitoring carbs in the meals you eat is the first step in carb counting. You're certainly aware that they're present in bread, spaghetti, and cake, but did you know that they're also present in leafy greens, yogurt, and beans?

Carbohydrates are often found in foods like salad dressing, pasta sauce, and protein bars, too. You should be aware of the foods that are primarily made up of carbs. You must know how to differentiate between protein-rich, fat-rich, and carbs-rich foods.

You must refrain from eating foods that are filled with empty carbs. Instead, eat those that have nutrients and fiber in them.

<u>Examples of foods high in fiber are:</u>

- Lentils
- Fruits
- Vegetables
- Oats
- Beans

Glycemic Index and Diabetes

If you have diabetes, you are well aware that carbs cause your blood sugar to rise. Your blood sugar is largely determined by the overall amount of carbs you ingest at a meal or snack. However, the meal itself has an impact. A serving of white rice has the same impact as pure table sugar in terms of causing a rapid, high blood sugar increase. Lentils have a gradual, less dramatic effect.

Choosing good carb sources can help you manage your blood sugar and weight. Eating healthy carbohydrates has been linked to a lower risk of heart disease and certain malignancies, as well as a range of chronic illnesses, including diabetes.

The glycemic index (GI) is one way to choose foods. The glycemic index (GI) is a number that indicates how much a particular item raises blood sugar levels. Foods are rated on a scale of 0–100 and classed as low, medium, or high glycemic foods. The lower a food's GI, the less likely it is to alter your blood sugar levels.

Foods with a high GI aren't always unhealthy, but they should be consumed in moderation. Choose more whole foods and eat highly processed foods less frequently or in smaller amounts to reduce the glycemic index.

It's simple to use the glycemic index: eat meals with a low GI instead of a high GI (see below), and take it easy on the things in between.

- Most fruits and vegetables, legumes, minimally processed grains, pasta, low-fat dairy foods, and nuts have a low glycemic index (GI of 55 or below).
- White and sweet potatoes, corn, white rice, couscous, and breakfast cereals like Cream of Wheat and Mini-Wheats have a moderate glycemic index (GI 56 to 69).
- White bread, rice cakes, most crackers, bagels, cakes, doughnuts, croissants, and packaged morning cereals have a high glycemic index (GI of 70 or above).

The Plate Method

It's really easy to consume more than you require without even realizing it. The plate technique is a straightforward, visual way to ensure that you consume enough non-starchy veggies and lean protein while reducing your intake of higher-carb meals that have the greatest impact on your blood sugar.

Begin with a 9-inch dinner plate (about the size of a business envelope):

> Salad, green beans, broccoli, cauliflower, cabbage, and carrots can be used to fill half of the bowl.

> One quarter should be filled with lean protein such as chicken, turkey, beans, tofu, or eggs.

> Fill one-quarter of your plate with carbohydrate-rich meals. Grain, starchy vegetables (such as potatoes and peas), rice, pasta, beans, fruit, and yogurt are all high in carbohydrates. A cup of milk is also a carbohydrate food.

> Then, to accompany your meal, drink water or a low-calorie beverage such as unsweetened iced tea.

Portion Sizes

The size of a portion and the size of a serving are not necessarily the same. A serving is a set amount of food, such as one slice of bread or 8 ounces (1 cup) of milk, whereas a portion is the amount of food you choose to eat at one time.

Restaurant portions are now far greater than they were a few years ago. One entrée might serve three or four people. People who are provided with more food prefer to eat more. Thus, portion control is critical for weight and blood sugar management.

If you're eating out, pack half of your meal to take home so you may consume it later. Measure out snacks at home. Don't consume them directly from the bag or box. Keep the serving bowls out of reach at dinnertime to avoid the temptation to go back for seconds.

And, thanks to this useful guide, you'll always be able to estimate portion sizes:

> When you have diabetes, no meal is off bounds. The trick is to keep track of your quantities, eat in a balanced manner, and consume around the same amount of carbohydrates at each meal.

> These four pointers, as well as dish suggestions for breakfast, lunch, and dinner, might help you get started.

> To learn how different food affects your blood sugar levels, take a blood sugar test.

> Stick to a specific carbohydrate gram count per meal. This is usually 45-75 grams three times per day.

In each meal, make sure to balance carbs, fiber, and protein. If you utilize the plate approach, this is simple. Half of your plate should be veggies, a quarter should be a carb like brown rice, black beans, or whole-wheat pasta, and the remaining quarter should be a healthy protein like chicken breast, fish, lean meat, or tofu. Depending on your carb goal for the meal, add a small piece of fruit and some low-fat or fat-free milk or yogurt.

Consume healthy fats from nuts, avocados, salmon, olives, and other plants. Saturated fats can be found in beef, butter, cheese, and other dairy products. Coconut, despite being a plant, contains saturated fat.

Recipes

Mediterranean Low Carb Broccoli Salad

Broccoli, artichoke hearts, sun-dried tomatoes, and onions are among the non-starchy veggies included in this salad. These meals are high in fiber, making you feel fuller for a longer period. Olives and olive oil provide heart-healthy fats, making this a heart-healthy option. According to the American Heart Association (AHA), olives and olive oil are high in monounsaturated fat, which helps lessen your risk of heart disease. According to the Centers for Disease Control and Prevention (CDC), diabetes doubles your risk of heart disease, hence monounsaturated fats should be prioritized in your diabetes diet.

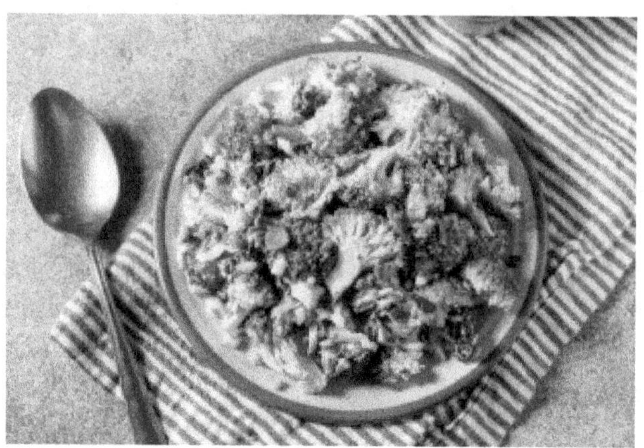

Ingredients

FOR THE SALAD:

- ✓ 5 cups broccoli, cut into small pieces

- ✓ ½ cup artichoke hearts, sliced and marinated in olive oil

- ✓ ½ cup sun-dried tomatoes, chopped (75g)

✓ ½ cup pitted Kalamata olives, halved

✓ 1/3 cup red onion, diced

✓ ¼ cup roasted salted sunflower seeds

FOR THE DRESSING:

✓ 2 cups Plain non-fat Greek yogurt

✓ Zest and juice of 1 large lemon

✓ 4 tsp monk fruit

✓ 1 tsp oregano

✓ 1 tsp garlic, minced

✓ 1 tsp dried ground basil

✓ 1 tsp dried ground thyme

✓ 1 tsp sea salt

✓ Pepper, to taste

✓ 2 tbsp oil from the jar of sun-dried tomatoes

Instructions

✓ Combine all of the dressing ingredients in a medium mixing bowl.

✓ Toss the broccoli with the dressing and toss well to coat.

✓ Cover and chill for at least 2 hours, preferably overnight, to allow the broccoli to absorb the dressing and develop flavor.

✓ Serve

Chicken Veggie Stir Fry

Stir-fries make it simple to prepare a diabetic-friendly meal. Carrots, broccoli, zucchini, and green onions are among the diabetes-friendly vegetables in this recipe. It also includes chicken as a lean protein option. To reduce saturated fat and cholesterol, the American Diabetes Association (ADA) recommends purchasing chicken without the skin.

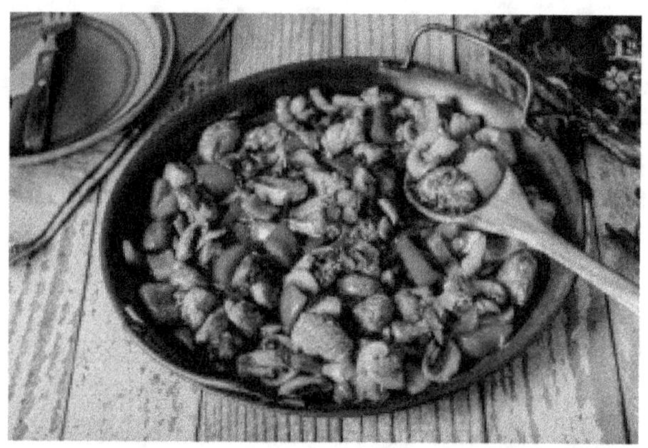

Salt, garlic, jalapeño, fresh ginger, lime, and reduced-sodium soy sauce add loads of flavor to this chicken and veggie dish. According to the US Food and Drug Administration (FDA), too much sodium, which is found in salt, can elevate blood pressure, raising the risk of heart disease.

Ingredients

- ✓ 2 tbsp soy sauce, divided

- ✓ 1 tbsp fresh ginger, minced

- ✓ 1 tbsp lemon juice, divided

- ✓ 2 tsp sesame oil, divided

- ✓ 1 lb skinless, boneless chicken breast

- ✓ 1 tbsp cold-pressed canola oil

✓ 2 carrots, cut into small rounds

✓ 2 cups broccoli florets

✓ 1 medium zucchini, cut in half lengthwise

✓ 4 garlic cloves, chopped

✓ 2 green onions, sliced

✓ 1 jalapeno pepper, sliced

✓ ½ cup fresh chopped basil

✓ ½ cup chopped cilantro, fresh

✓ Brown rice, optional

Instructions

✓ In a big zip-top plastic bag or dish, combine 1 tablespoon soy sauce, ginger, half a lime juice, and 1 teaspoon sesame oil.

✓ Refrigerate for 1 hour or up to 24 hours after adding the chicken pieces to the bag.

✓ Heat the oil in a big wok or nonstick skillet over medium-high heat when you're ready to prepare your stir fry.

✓ Stir in the chicken and the marinade for one minute.

✓ Stir in the carrots, broccoli, zucchini, garlic, green onions, and jalapeño pepper for 7 minutes more, or until the chicken is cooked through and the vegetables are crisp-tender.

✓ Combine the remaining 1 tablespoon soy sauce, the remaining lime juice, and the remaining sesame oil in a large mixing bowl.

✓ Stir in the basil and cilantro just before serving.

✓ As preferred, serve with brown rice.

Lentil Tacos

Green lentils, vegetable broth, diced tomatoes, green chilies, yellow onion, garlic, cilantro, lime, and a variety of spices are all used in these meatless tacos. The following spices are used: cumin, chili powder, ancho chili powder, paprika, and cayenne pepper. Using pulses like lentils instead of standard taco starches like rice may decrease sugar digestion, decreasing blood sugar levels in the long run.

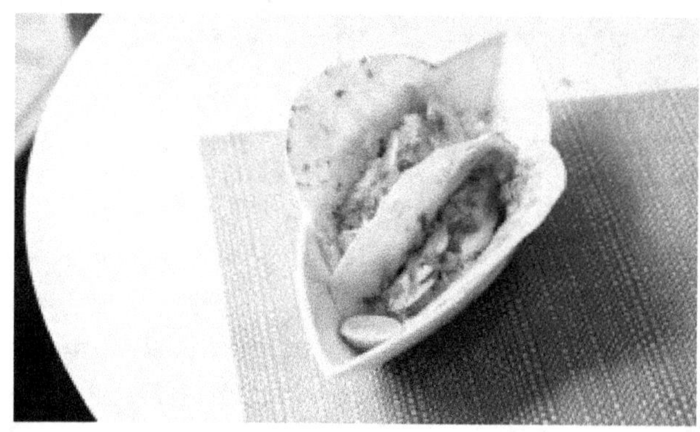

Ingredients

✓ 1 cup green lentils, rinsed

✓ 4 cups vegetable broth

✓ 1 can diced tomatoes and green chilies

✓ 1 tbsp olive oil

✓ 1 cup chopped yellow onion

✓ 3 tsp minced garlic

✓ 3 tsp ground cumin

✓ 1 tsp chili powder

✓ 1 tsp ancho chili powder

✓ 2 tsp paprika

✓ Salt and freshly ground black pepper, to taste

✓ 3 tbsp chopped fresh cilantro

✓ 1 tbsp fresh lime juice

For serving

✓ Corn tortillas or crisp taco shells, lettuce, cheese, tomatoes (for serving)

Instructions

✓ In a 5.-6.-quart slow cooker, combine the lentils, broth, olive oil, tomatoes, onions, garlic, chili powders, and paprika. Season with salt and pepper.

✓ Cover and cook on high for 3–4 hours, or low for 7–8 hours.

✓ Add the cilantro and lime juice and mix well.

✓ Warm tortillas with toppings should be served for the best taste.

Lemon Garlic Salmon

According to the American Heart Association, rich fish like baked salmon in this recipe is a good source of omega-3 polyunsaturated fatty acids. If you have Type 2 diabetes, meals high in omega-3 fatty acids may help lower your risk of problems such as heart disease and stroke. Salmon is baked with healthful, fragrant ingredients including lemons, lemon zest, garlic cloves, olive oil, and fresh parsley in this dish.

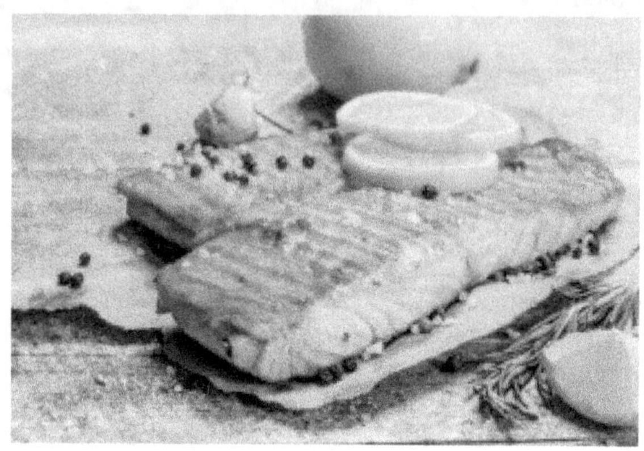

Ingredients

- ✓ ½ pound salmon fillet
- ✓ 3 medium lemons, sliced
- ✓ 2 tsp lemon zest
- ✓ 4 garlic cloves, minced
- ✓ 2 tbsp extra virgin olive oil
- ✓ 1 tsp kosher salt
- ✓ ½ tsp freshly ground black pepper
- ✓ Chopped fresh parsley

Instructions

✓ Preheat the oven to 400°F and oil a baking dish large enough to hold all of the salmon pieces.

✓ In a mixing bowl, combine the lemon juice, garlic, oil, salt, and pepper.

✓ Fill a Ziploc bag with the salmon fillets and the lemon marinade.

✓ Seal the bag and move the salmon pieces around to evenly coat them with the marinade.

✓ Allow for at least 30 minutes of marinating time.

✓ Layer the lemon slices into your prepared plate, then top with the salmon.

✓ Bake the salmon for 12-15 minutes, or until it is fully cooked.

✓ The thickness of your salmon will determine how long it takes to cook.

✓ After that, place a couple of slices of lemon on top of the grilled salmon and turn the oven to broil.

✓ Broil for 3 minutes, or until golden and crisp on top.

✓ Remove from the oven and sprinkle with parsley before serving.

Zucchini Lasagna

Traditional lasagna is high in calories, carbohydrates, and saturated fat, making it a poor choice for Type 2 diabetics. This recipe, however, uses zucchini instead of pasta to drastically reduce carbs and calories without sacrificing flavor.

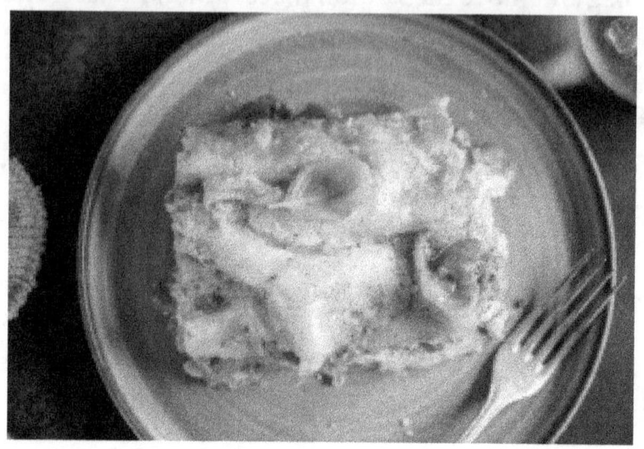

Zucchini provides a lot of nutrients. One medium zucchini, for example, has 35 grams of vitamin C, making it a great source of vitamin. Many persons with Type 2 diabetes may be deficient in this antioxidant, possibly due to high levels of oxidative stress caused by anomalies in blood sugar metabolism.

Ingredients

- ✓ 15 oz ground beef

- ✓ 2 medium zucchinis

- ✓ 4 medium onion

- ✓ 2 garlic cloves

- ✓ 1 green chili

- ✓ 2 tomatoes

- ✓ 5 oz mushrooms

- ✓ 1 cup Knorr chicken bouillon

- ✓ 1 cup shredded mozzarella

- ✓ 1 tsp paprika

✓ 1 tsp dried thyme

✓ 1 tsp dried basil

✓ Salt and pepper, to taste

Instructions

✓ Cut the zucchini into 12-inch (1-cm) pieces with a julienne peeler. Set aside for 10 minutes after lightly seasoning with salt.

✓ Using a paper towel, blot the zucchini slices. Grill or broil them for 3 minutes at high heat in the oven.

✓ Place the zucchini on paper towels after grilling or broiling (you want to get as much of the liquid out as possible).

✓ Make an X insertion in the top of the tomatoes by cutting off the ends. Place in boiling water for a few minutes, then drain and peel off the skin with cool water. Alternatively, canned tomatoes could be utilized.

✓ Onions, garlic, chili, skinned tomatoes, and mushrooms should be roughly chopped.

✓ In a deep skillet, coat with cooking spray and sauté the garlic, onion, and chili for 1 minute.

✓ In the same skillet, add the tomatoes and mushrooms and cook for a further 4 minutes.

✓ Remove them from the heat and set them aside.

✓ In the same skillet as the vegetables, sauté the meat with the paprika until fully cooked.

✓ Return the vegetables to the skillet, then add the remaining spices and chicken bouillon.

✓ Allow the sauce to boil on low heat for 25 minutes.

✓ Preheat the oven to 375 degrees Fahrenheit (190 C).

✓ Use 1/3 of the zucchini to construct a layer in the bottom of a small baking tray lined with parchment paper. 1/3 of the meat sauce should be on top.

✓ Continue with another layer of zucchini until you've used up all of the sauce and zucchini.

✓ Bake for 35 minutes with shredded mozzarella on top.

✓ Remove the lasagna from the oven and set it aside for 10 minutes to cool before serving.

Cauliflower Tacos

Try these roasted cauliflower tacos for a vegetarian supper. The taco filling is made up of heart-healthy olive oil and non-starchy cauliflower cooked in taco spice.

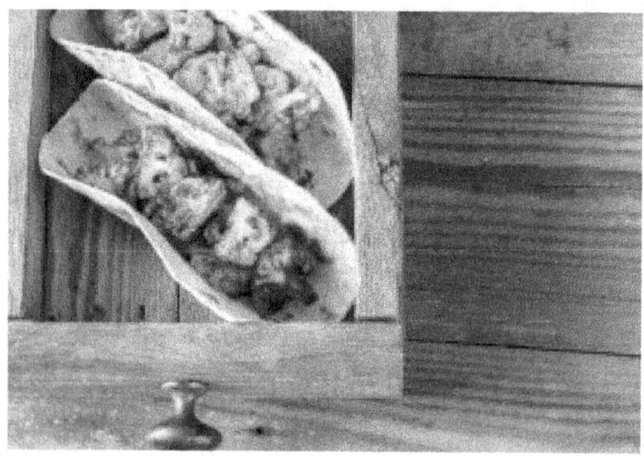

It's then topped with a homemade avocado lime sauce, which offers a bit of plant-based protein and healthy fats for satiety. To cut down on carbs, serve in tortillas or lettuce wraps. Pickled red onions, chopped cilantro, and a smidgeon of queso fresco or feta cheese on top (optional).

Ingredients

- ✓ 1 head of medium cauliflower
- ✓ 1 tbsp olive oil
- ✓ 2 tsp taco seasoning

Avocado Lime Sauce

- ✓ 1 avocado
- ✓ 1 fresh lemon juice and zest
- ✓ 1 tsp kosher salt

For serving

- ✓ Tortillas
- ✓ Feta cheese (optional)
- ✓ Chopped cilantro (optional)

Instructions

Roast Cauliflower

- ✓ Preheat oven to 425 degrees.
- ✓ Cauliflower should be cut into florets.
- ✓ Drizzle olive oil over cauliflower and season with taco seasoning.
- ✓ Spread out on a large baking sheet after tossing to evenly coat with seasonings.

✓ If necessary, divide the cauliflower between two pans to avoid overcrowding and ensure optimal roasting.

✓ Roast for 30-40 minutes, flipping once during the cooking duration, until soft and golden.

Make Avocado Lime Sauce

✓ In a blender or tiny food processor, mash ripe avocado.

✓ In a food processor, combine fresh lime juice, lime zest, and salt; process until smooth and creamy, scraping down sides as needed.

✓ If your sauce needs to be thinned, add 1 tablespoon of cold water.

Assemble

✓ Place roasted cauliflower onto a tortilla or lettuce wrap to make Cauliflower Tacos.

✓ Drizzle with avocado sauce and, if desired, garnish with pickled red onions, cilantro, and cheese.

Slow Cooker Chicken Noodle Soup

Skinless chicken breasts, low-sodium chicken broth, garlic, onion, carrots, celery, and a variety of herbs are combined in this hearty chicken noodle soup. It also substitutes zucchini for spaghetti noodles. It's low-carb because there are no noodles, making it an excellent alternative for someone limiting their carb consumption.

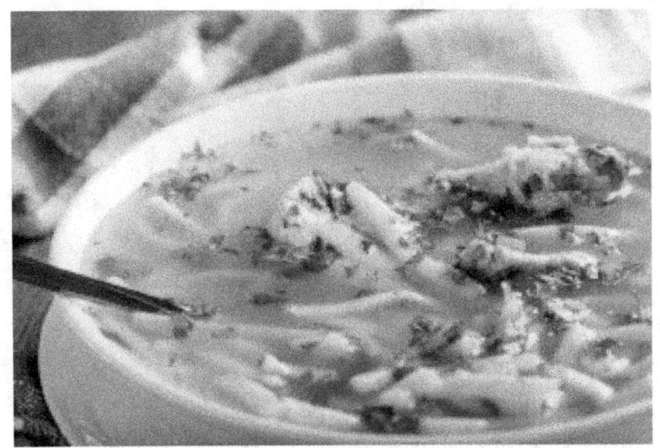

Ingredients

- ✓ 1 lb boneless, skinless chicken breasts

- ✓ 1 tsp sea salt (even more if needed)

- ✓ 1 tsp ground black pepper

- ✓ 3 cloves garlic, minced

- ✓ 1 medium yellow onion, diced

- ✓ 4 medium carrots, sliced

- ✓ 2 stalks celery, sliced

- ✓ 6 cups low sodium chicken broth

- ✓ 2 bay leaf

- ✓ 2 medium zucchinis, cut in a spiral shape

- ✓ 1 tsp fresh thyme

- ✓ 1 tsp fresh rosemary

- ✓ 1 tbsp freshly squeezed lemon juice (approx. 1 tbsp)

✓ 2 tbsp fresh parsley, chopped

Instructions

✓ Season the chicken with salt and pepper to taste.

✓ In a slow cooker, place the seasoned chicken.

✓ Stir together the garlic, onion, carrots, celery, and chicken stock.

✓ Cover and simmer for 6-8 hours on low heat or 4-5 hours on high heat, or until the chicken is cooked through and the vegetables are soft.

✓ Using two forks, shred the cooked chicken from the slow cooker.

✓ Stir in the spiralized zucchini noodles, thyme, and rosemary until well combined.

✓ Cook for a further 8-10 minutes on low heat, or until the zucchini is largely tender, covered in the slow cooker.

✓ Combine the lemon juice and parsley in a mixing bowl.

Easy Quinoa Salad

Don't be intimidated by quinoa. It's quite simple to prepare. Quinoa is one of my favorite grains to cook with because it is nutritious, hearty, and high in protein. I like to prepare the quinoa ahead of time so that the salad comes together quickly. Cooked quinoa can be stored in the refrigerator for up to one week. This quinoa salad is also gluten-free and vegan. It's a delicious and nutritious lunch, supper, or side dish for any meal. This easy quinoa salad is very easy to prepare and diabetic friendly, too. It has very few carbs that have a low glycemic index, too.

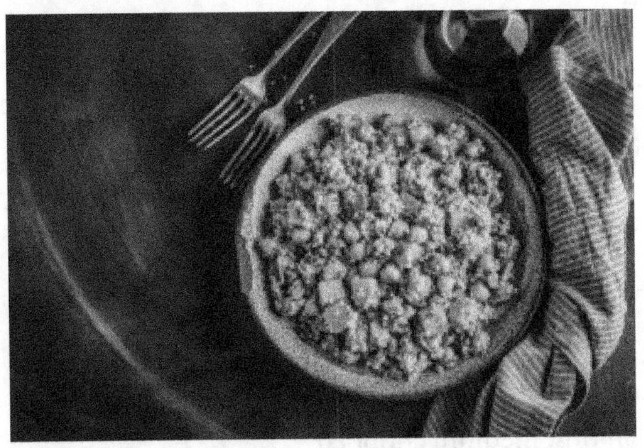

You can add shredded chicken, chickpeas, or white beans to make the quinoa salad more of a main dish.

The ideal day to eat this quinoa salad is the day it's made, but sometimes the leftovers are fine the next day as well. The avocado will not brown because of the lemon in the dressing. If you wish to make the salad ahead of time, combine everything except the avocado and the dressing together. When you're ready to dine, add the avocado and dressing, and the salad will be very fresh.

Ingredients

For the Dressing

> ½ cup extra virgin olive oil

> 2 cloves garlic, minced

> 2 tbsp lime juice or 1 large lemon

> 1 tbsp golden balsamic vinegar

> 1 tsp honey or pure maple syrup

> Black pepper and kosher salt, to taste

For the Salad

> 2 cup cold cooked quinoa

> 2 cups medium spinach leaves, chopped

> ½ cup cucumber, chopped

> 1 cup cherry tomatoes, sliced

> 1 large ripe avocado, pitted, peeled, and chopped finely

> 2 green onions, medium chopped

> Freshly ground black pepper and kosher salt, to taste

Instructions

> Make the dressing first. Whisk together the olive oil, garlic, lemon juice, vinegar, maple syrup or honey, salt, and pepper in a small bowl or jar. Remove from the equation.

> Combine the quinoa, spinach, cucumber, tomatoes, avocado, and green onions in a large mixing basin.

> Drizzle the dressing over the salad and gently mix until it is evenly distributed.

> Season the salad with salt and pepper.

> Serve.

SUMMARY

Many people these days are facing the most common disease that is diabetes. In this book, every aspect and detail of diabetes has been shared with you so you can learn about the silent killer that diabetes mellitus is. From the introduction of diabetes, types, reversal to dietary guidelines all have been covered in detail. The main two types of diabetes that are Type 1 Diabetes and Type 2 Diabetes have been discussed along with their risk factors, causes, etiology, and prevention. Then, in the next chapters, you have learned about the reversal of each type of diabetes with all the pros and cons of each method used for treating these conditions. By now, you are aware of all the things and terminologies related to this disease that affects millions of people. As it is a very common disease, its complications are also very diverse. It almost affects every organ of the human body. All the complications related to diabetes Type 1 and Type 2 are mentioned in detail for your convenience. In the last chapter, you have learned in detail how to manage and control your diabetes with the help of diet. All dietary guidelines are provided so you can easily help yourself or your loved ones to fight this grave disease. Many recipes and meals have also been provided with the instructions and method of preparation so you can easily prepare them at home and manage your diabetes easily.

Don't miss out!

Visit the website below and you can sign up to receive emails whenever Dr. Robertino Bedenian publishes a new book. There's no charge and no obligation.

https://books2read.com/r/B-A-YQGQ-AHKUC

BOOKS 2 READ

Connecting independent readers to independent writers.

Also by Dr. Robertino Bedenian

Fitness Over 60 For Women – How to Stay Fit And Healthy As You Age

Does Back Pain Go Away? 10 Answers To The Most Acute Back Pain Issues

Massage Bible - A Beginners Guide To Western And Eastern Massage Therapy

Going Vegan - How To Vegan Without Going Crazy

Chiropraktik - Was Steckt Eigentlich Dahinter?

Massagen: Ein Überblick Über Westliche Und Östliche Massagetechniken

Natuerlich Abnehmen, Schlank Und Endlich Fit Sein

P.S. Ich Liebe Dich: Wenn Liebe So Einfach Wäre

Was Tun Bei Rückenschmerzen, Bandscheibenvorfall Und Ischiasschmerzen: 10 Antworten Zu Den Häufigsten Fragen Bei Rückenschmerzen

Was Tun Gegen Schlafapnoe, Schlafstörungen Und Schnarchen

Self-Help Books for Women – How to Overcome Depression, Anxiety, Divorce, Addiction, and Trauma

Diabetes How to Help: Everything You Need to Know About Diabetes Type 1 and Type 2

Diet and Workout Planner: How to Stay Healthy and Get Fit for Life

Everything I Know About Love

The Sleep Easy Solution Book: How to Stop Sleep Apnea, Snoring, and Sleep Disorders

Your Super Gut Feeling Restored – How to Restore Your Life Energy and Overall Health from The Inside Out

Watch for more at https://booksummarypublishing.com.

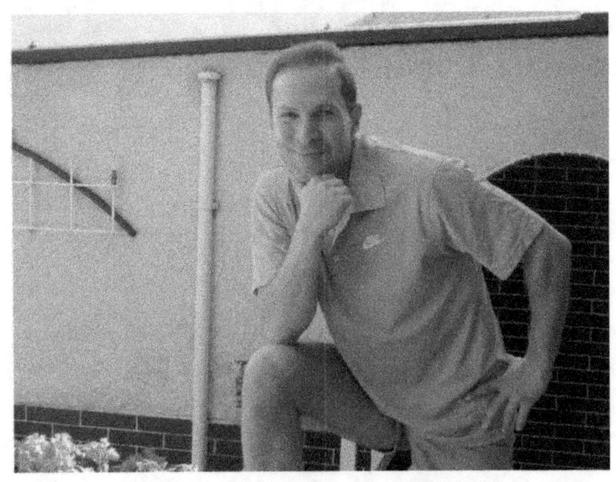

About the Author

Dr. Robertino Bedenian is a qualified fitness instructor accredited by the German Olympic Committee, a health and nutrition expert, and the author of several books on diet, health, and fitness!

For more than twenty years he has been a fitness coach at the sports university teaching aerobics, back gymnastics, stretching, high-intensity interval training (HIIT), power gymnastics, and athletic sports.

On his website, he has published more than 300 articles about the vegan lifestyle covering diet and health recommendations, detoxication programs, fitness guidelines, and disease-related topics. He is part of a family with an orthopedic surgeon, a physical therapist, an osteopath, and an alternative practitioner.

He is also the founder of the brand "**Going Vegan**" selling high-quality supplements for optimal health.

You are more than welcome to check his website for more details: https://goingveganhealthbenefits.com.

His brand has been awarded continuously with 5-star feedback by customers for its outstanding product quality.

Dr. Bedenian is also the founder of the book company "**Book Summary Publishing**" publishing summaries and workbooks of Amazon #1 bestselling non-fiction books.

If you want to learn more about the summaries and workbooks that he has published so far, please visit his website:

https://booksummarypublishing.com
Read more at https://booksummarypublishing.com.